ABOUT THE AUTHOR

Brian Livesley MD FRCP has been committed whole-time to the National Health Service since qualifying in Leeds in 1960. After several years wide experience in general medicine he became the Harvey Research Fellow at King's College Hospital where he devised and established new laboratory and clinical techniques for the study of ischaemic heart disease. In 1973, as consultant geriatrician, he introduced then new clinical audit procedures to raise the standard of care of elderly people in hospital and community. As a result of this and his other researches and teaching he was invited to professorial chairs abroad which he declined. In 1988, he took up post as the University of London's Professor in the Care of the Elderly and became based at Chelsea & Westminster Hospital, London, where he developed a 'leading edge' service for elderly people reported by the King's Fund and copied internationally. His dual-accredited specialist registrar training programme became the national norm. He developed one of the first palliative care services for non-cancer patients. He was appointed Emeritus Professor in the Care of the Elderly at Imperial College, London University in 2003 'to mark a distinguished career'. Since 2001 he has worked by invitation as a consultant forensic physician with National Police Constabularies and Coroner's Offices. He is a medical historian and was Master of the Society of Apothecaries in 2005-2006.

D1642692

The Dying Keats

A CASE FOR EUTHANASIA?

To Stuart

a very good friend

Bri

BRIAN LIVESLEY

Emeritus Professor in the Care of the Elderly,
Imperial College, London University

Matador
5 Weir Road
Kibworth Beauchamp
Leicester LE8 0LQ, UK
Tel: (+44) 116 279 2299
Email: books@troubador.co.uk
Web: www.troubador.co.uk/matador

ISBN 978-1848761-711

A Cataloguing-in-Publication (CIP) catalogue record for this book
is available from the British Library.

Cover: 'The Dying Keats' © City of London, Keats House.

Typeset in 11pt Book Antiqua by Troubador Publishing Ltd, Leicester, UK

Matador is an imprint of Troubador Publishing Ltd

Printed in Great Britain by the MPG Books Group, Bodmin and King's Lynn

'The Dying Keats' picture on the front cover has been reproduced by kind permission of Keats House. It is usually known as 'John Keats on his death-bed' and was drawn in ink by Joseph Severn. Underneath it Severn had written, '28 Janr. [1821] 3 o'clock mng. Drawn to keep me awake – a deadly sweat was on him all this night.' Keats died 25 days later.

FOREWORD

As failures in medical care lead to repeated cries for the legalisation of euthanasia, the avoidable and prolonged suffering John Keats endured before he died is particularly relevant today. Several factors contributed to his distress. He was the first to recognise he would die from tuberculosis; he was repeatedly troubled by severe criticism of his poetry; and, crucially during the last three months of what he described as 'this posthumous life of mine', he was constantly denied relief from his suffering despite the availability of opium.

This publication raises several questions. It is hoped that it will stimulate an appropriate debate and lead to a better recognition by all professionals at the bedside that dying is a clinical diagnosis which requires action. Once this is understood, the needs of patients and their relatives can be earlier and more appropriately addressed. Those who are dying should not have to undergo the "Keatsian experience". They, as well as their relatives and friends, should know that palliative care properly delivered can mean the end of unendurable distress in life's last weeks, days, and hours. Indeed, no person dying in the United Kingdom today should have to seek legalised euthanasia to be comfortable as they approach the end of their life.

Since 1969 the John Keats' Biennial Memorial Lecture has been supported in London by Guy's Hospital, the Worshipful Society of Apothecaries, and the Royal College of Surgeons of England, but the link these organisations have with Keats may not be widely known.

After leaving school in 1810, Keats began a five years' apothecary apprenticeship in Edmonton. Then in 1815 he began training in surgical practice at Guy's Hospital and, a year later, after examination at the Worshipful Society of Apothecaries in London's Blackfriars, he qualified as an apothecary. As is well known, he left clinical practice to write poetry. John Keats died, at the age of 25, on the 23rd February 1821 — hence the February date for his memorial lectures.

Those who have read and commented on this twentieth biennial Keats' memorial lecture know who they are and of my gratitude. They have no responsibility for any of the comments made, errors committed, or opinions expressed — all are mine.

Should there be any profits after publication these will go to the Society of Apothecaries to help fund medical students to study one of 'the medical humanities' in their final year.

Brian Livesley
February 2009

On First Looking into Chapman's Homer
by John Keats

Much have I travell'd in the realms of gold,
And many goodly states and kingdoms seen;
Round many western islands have I been
Which bards in fealty to Apollo hold.
Oft of one wide expanse had I been told
That deep-brow'd Homer ruled as his demesne;
Yet did I never breathe its pure serene
Till I heard Chapman speak out loud and bold:
Then felt I like some watcher of the skies
When a new planet swims into his ken;
Or like stout Cortez when with eagle eyes
He star'd at the Pacific and–all his men
Look'd at each other with a wild surmise–
Silent, upon a peak in Darien. [1,2,3,4]

… and having written this, arguably his most famously admired and curiously 'anagrammatic sonnet',[5] John Keats broke into English history. It was 1816; exactly 200 years after Chapman had translated the Iliad.[6] After reading Keats' sonnet for the first time, his friend Joseph Severn said 'I confess that at that moment I also felt like Cortez when he stared at the Pacific … I knew the first works of Burns and of Byron, and they could not compare with my friend as regards these first attempts. And even Chatterton seemed to me inferior in the poetical fire ....'[7]

Within five years Keats was dying. According to Shelley and Byron his death was the result of repeated severe criticism of his poetry by John Gibson Lockhart. Indeed, on his sick-bed, Keats told another of his friends, John Reynolds, 'If I die, you must ruin Lockhart'[!][8]

So what was it about Keats' poetry that had created such adversity and did it hasten his death? Was it simply his inverted poetic style? By that, what do I mean?

In Keats' poetry the action, the descriptive, occurs not only at the end of line and verse but also at the poem's end[9]—what journalists call 'the delayed drop'. For example not ... 'I have travell'd much in golden realms' but capturing the reader's attention with the necessary pauses associated with inversions ... 'much have I travell'd ... in the realms of gold' [...] 'Yet did I never breathe its pure serene / Till I heard Chapman speak out loud and bold...' ... but more about this later.

T.E. Lawrence, of Arabia fame, 'Reflecting on what he regarded as the exaggerated protraction of the final events in Homer's Odyssey, ...' commented on '...the tedious delay of the climax through ten books ...'[10] So what lit up Keats' sense of wonder about Chapman's Homer? Moreover, would Keats have discovered the breadth and depth of his own poetic imagination and his melancholic musings about death without the stimulus of Chapman?

To determine this we need briefly to consider a few lines from other translations available at that time; while bearing in mind that the subject of Homer's Iliad is 'anger, Achilles' anger', his uncontrollable anger, indeed, his consuming rage. This was well described in the opening lines of this epic by Calchas (the famous Greek soothsayer whose curses open the Iliad[11] and who had seen that Troy would not be defeated if Achilles did not fight with the Greeks). Indeed, Achilles' anger was the driving force within the story of the Trojan War. Without this, as Manguel has commented, there would be no story.[12]

Chapman's 1616 translation, with the title page showing Achilles on the left and Hector on the right, opens the Iliad with, 'Achilles' baneful wrath – resound, O goddess – that impos'd / Infinite sorrows on the Greeks/'; whereas, in 1715, Thomas Ticknell had given Achilles a '...fatal wrath, whence discord rose' and, then Alexander Pope, who in his correspondence regarded his translation of Homer as a 'drudge',[13] simply wrote 'Achilles' wrath, whence Discord rose/That brought the Sons of Greece unnumber'd Woes,' but then Pope limps off the line with ... 'O Goddess sing' and his final version of 1736 was no better. Whereas, Cowper's 1791 version written in rivalry with Pope reads 'Achilles sing, O Goddess! Peleus son; his wrath pernicious....'

It appears to me, as it apparently did to Keats, that when read out loud, as his friend Cowden Clarke had done for Keats that October evening in 1816,[14] Chapman's—'Achilles' baneful wrath–resound...' (the 'bane' part referring to an archaic Old English word for death) speaks out loud and bold. It paves the way for readers even now to be 'watchers from the skies' as the epic narrative unfolds the moods of men and shows the violent deaths of many including Hector. Furthermore, as Slote has stated, compared with Pope's translation using 10 syllable lines of closed couplets, Chapman's open lines of 14 syllables require a longer, more irregular and racy breath. This, together with his more colourful and exciting language carries the reader forward at a rousing pace; and it shows Achilles, before he died, as a figure of noble principles, who could convert his anger, his great and awesome rage, resentment, and hostility into reconciliation with Agamemnon. Need one say more, except to ask could Keats do the same with Lockhart?

So much has been written about Keats that it is difficult for anyone to be original, but a summary may be helpful, particularly if we focus on his botanical knowledge.

It is well known that Keats took an apothecary apprenticeship in Edmonton, just outside London. During this he would accumulate extensive experience in the medicinal properties of many herbs. After the licensing Apothecaries Act of 1815, Guy's was the only institution capable of providing all the medical teaching required for the Society's diploma. In 1816, and in addition to his surgical training at Guy's, Keats attended the herborising excursions of William Salisbury. Salisbury was the favoured botany teacher at Guy's Hospital and his botanical lessons competed with the time consuming and costly excursions of the Society of Apothecaries. On the 25th June that year, Alexander Marcet, a physician at Guy's and a Fellow of the Royal Society, on whose chemistry course Keats had enrolled, read a paper 'On the Medicinal Properties of Stramonium'.[15] The effects of Stramonium [or datura as it is more widely known] have been described as 'a living dream: consciousness falls in and out, people who don't exist or are miles away are conversed with.'[16] It is, perhaps, in relation to Keats' failed and much criticised poem *Endymion* we need to reflect that the effects of datura and other herbals can last for days. On the 25th July 1816 — having completed his botanical course, and producing evidence from Guy's that he had also attended the necessary courses in anatomy, physiology, chemistry and *materia medica* — Keats sat the Apothecaries' diploma examination.[17] Pictures of herbs in the Society of Apothecaries' archives (including datura, poppy, and hemlock) are some of those that were used during the examination to test the candidates' knowledge.

While others were failed, Keats passed at his first attempt and became one of the new generation of apothecaries. After opting out of a medical career,

5

his interest in botany and gardening continued throughout his brief life.[18] Indeed, only five years later, on his deathbed in Rome in 1821, he told Joseph Severn 'perhaps the only happiness I have had in the world—has been the silent growth of flowers.'[19]

But Keats' interest in botany found other expressions. In his ode *To a Nightingale* he states:

> My heart aches, and a drowsy numbness pains
> My sense, as though of hemlock I had drunk,
> Or emptied some dull opiate to the drains
> One minute past, and Lethe-wards[20] had sunk:
> ...
> O for a draught of vintage that hath been
> Cool'd a long age in the deep-delvèd earth,
> Tasting of Flora and the country green, ...
> ...
> O for a beaker full of warm South,
> Full of the true, the blissful Hippocrene,[21]
> With beaded bubbles winking at the brim,[22]
> And purple-stainèd mouth;
> That I might drink, and leave the world unseen,
> And with thee fade away into the forest dim.

We should note that drinking 'Hippocrene' water was supposed to bring forth poetic inspiration.

'The purple-stainèd mouth' describes the stain from drinking the reddish purple 'blood' obtained from the sap of St. John's wort used to protect the drinker from fairy trickery.[23]

Hemlock was alleged to have wide curative properties. But, because of the death of Socrates, its lethal properties are better known.[24] Few have considered, however, what took place *before* Socrates drank his cup, when he first wanted to offer a libation to the gods, but was told by his keeper, 'We only prepare, Socrates, just so much as we deem enough.'[25] ... It is not widely known that a judicious dose of hemlock can act simply like a narcotic. This use was well known at and after Keats' time.[26] Indeed, as recently as seven years ago, hemlock was described as being responsible for a reversible coma in the case of a Scotsman, a brain surgeon, who was reported to have eaten some while hill walking in the north of Scotland;[27] presumably because of its similarity to wild parsley or celery.[28]

There is no doubt that Keats was well aware of the effects on the mind of the variety of herbals that were so easily obtainable from the fields, but did he use them? There is certainly evidence that he used opium secretly; as others did socially until the late nineteenth century when physicians began speaking out against its regular use.

It seems that Keats first acquired a taste for opium in March 1819 after he had been hit in the eye with a cricket ball. His friend Brown, in whose house he was living, gave him some as a palliative. Despite his painful eye injury he slept late into the following morning, which is unusual after such trauma. A few weeks later he wrote his ode *To a*

Nightingale. His low spirits after the recent death of his brother, Tom, adds a more poignant perception to aspects of this Ode, which reads...

> Darkling I listen; and for many a time
> I have been half in love with easeful Death,
> Call'd him soft names in many a musèd rhyme,
> To take into the air my quiet breath;
> Now more than ever seems it rich to die,
> To cease upon the midnight with no pain,
> While thou art pouring forth thy soul abroad
> In such an ecstasy!
> Still wouldst thou sing, and I have ears in vain
> To thy high requiem become a sod.

And his ode *Indolence* a few weeks later reads:

> ... Ripe was the drowsy hour;
> The blissful cloud of summer-indolence
> Benumb'd my eyes; my pulse grew less and less;[29]
> Pain had no sting,[30] and pleasure's wreath no
> flower:
> O, why did ye not melt, and leave my sense
> Unhaunted quite of all but – nothingness?

We should note that slowing of the pulse is one of the effects of opium and an initial effect of hemlock.

Readers of Keats' ode *On a Grecian Urn* written in the same year, 1819, will find it has a similar dreamy[31] slow pace. As Lloyd has stated recently, 'For Keats, the "materials" of poetry are language and bodily sensation, which feed the imagination and provide its transforming energy.'[32]

Moreover, in *The fall of Hyperion* (also 1819), subtitled *A Dream*, Keats records:

… thereby
Stood a cool vessel of transparent juice ....
That full draught is parent of my theme. ….
Among the fragrant husks and berries crush'd,
Upon the grass I struggled hard against
The domineering potion; but in vain:
The cloudy swoon came on, and down I sank
Like a Silenus[33] on an antique vase.
How long I slumber'd 'tis a chance to guess.
When sense of life return'd, I started up
As if with wings; but the fair trees were gone,
The mossy mound and arbour were no more: ….

It may be difficult to find more compelling evidence of Keats' personal use of herbal medicines and unnecessary; since at this time Brown recorded '… he began to be reckless of health. Among other proofs of recklessness, he was secretly taking at times, a few drops of laudanum to keep up his spirits. It was discovered by accident, and, without delay, revealed to me.'[34,35]

Laudanum can induce a slowed pulse rate and a relaxed clouding of consciousness as well as hallucinations which could facilitate poetic inspiration, as Coleridge and others discovered. But today some may defend their hero by contending Keats merely used his awareness of the actions of botanical drugs within his poetic imagination rather than by experiencing the use of the drugs themselves. As was pointed out by Hayter 40 years ago,[36] there is no *absolute* evidence that Keats ever tasted laudanum before the winter of 1819-1820, by which time he had written all his important poetry, but she failed to recognise the significance of its major constituent, opium, given to Keats several months earlier in March 1819. This controversy is not my major thesis but rather that Keats had knowledge and access to such preparations which later were completely denied him as he lay dying in severe distress in Rome.

So what had happened to our young poet during the few years he poured out some of the best of English poetry and did criticism hasten his illness and death?

With now recognised, but at the time, hidden editorial support from Walter Scott and at monthly intervals from the first volume of *Blackwood's Edinburgh Magazine*, Keats' poetry was repeatedly and witheringly criticised by John Gibson Lockhart. He was a year older than Keats and had discovered from Benjamin Bailey, another of Keats' friends, that the poet had been a dresser at Guy's having already served a five years' apothecary apprenticeship. Keats knew his weak point was his poem *Endymion*. Lockhart picked on this in his review, written in 1818 under the sneering heading 'The Cockney School of Poetry' while using the protective pen-name 'Z'. He wrote, 'Whether Mr.

John had been sent home with a diuretic or composing draught to some patient far gone in the poetical mania, we have not heard. This much is certain, that he has caught the infection. For some time we were in hopes that he might get off with a violent fit or two, but of late the symptoms are terrible. The frenzy of the Poems was bad enough in its way; but it did not alarm us half so seriously as the calm, settled, imperturbable drivelling-idiocy of Endymion', and Lockhart concluded, 'It is a better and a wiser thing to be a starved apothecary than a starved poet; so back to the shop, Mr. John, "back to the plasters, pills and ointment boxes, &c." but for heaven's sake, young Sangrado, be a little more sparing of extentuatives and soporifics in your practice than you have been in your poetry.' [37]

Lockhart wrote but never published his own poems nor did he disclose the prose pieces he had written and published in various places.[38] In 1935, his biographer, Gilbert Macbeth, stated that Lockhart's articles about '… Keats especially, are not vindictive, but good-humoured; a tone of playful raillery is sustained throughout.'

'The satire [Macbeth adds] is of the sort that stings but does not rankle. ….'[39] Having just read Lockhart's words can we agree, especially when in the light of the fierceness of his criticisms he became known as 'The Scorpion'?[40]

Lockhart's comments about starvation and Sangrado were particularly biting. Keats had inscribed his poem *Endymion* to the memory of Thomas Chatterton, who Keats thought was second only to Shakespeare and who, rather than die of starvation, committed suicide by arsenic in 1779 at the young age of 17. Moreover, Lockhart's description of Keats as 'young Sangrado' referred to the literary figure, Dr Sangrado, who thought it a gross error to suppose that blood was necessary for life. He would repeatedly bleed his patients copiously replacing this loss by making them drink two or three pints of hot water every two hours until they died.[41]

Both Shelley and Byron stated that the contemptuous analysis of Keats' poetry was responsible for his death. Their opinions have to be doubted since a careful analysis made in 1934, entitled Keats and the periodicals of his time,[42] showed that from 1816-1821 of 30 listed reviews of his poetry '... eighteen were predominantly favourable, [only] four [including Lockhart's] definitely hostile, and the remainder either neutral or doubtful.'

One reason for such critical Scottish behaviour appears to relate to the established style of Scottish poetry, which had helped restore a sense of national pride after years of humiliation by the English,[43] let alone the Tory policies of the Scots opposing the radical attitudes of the Keats' literary circle.

Lockhart, Walter Scott, and others had grown up

with the 18th century Scottish life-breathing poetry of Allan Ramsay, Henry Erskine, Michael Bruce, Robert Fergusson, and others including Burns, whose biography Lockhart later wrote.[44] It can be misleading to quote from any person's poetic life but for me, despite fluent rhyming, the style of these Scots poets too often carries a repetitive ti-túm, ti-túm, ti-túm rhythm—which recalls ... the kind of pace ye gain ... striding o'er the heather! It is difficult to avoid the conclusion that Keats' poetic inversions provoked the envy and resentment of the Scots because—although their poets had previously copied the English iambic style used by Alexander Pope, George Crabbe, and the hymn writers such as William Cowper and Isaac Watts (the English Father of Hymnody whose works appeared in the Scottish Psalter)—the Scots had not discovered and developed the more resounding Keatsian style for themselves. Interestingly, Lockhart had difficulty preparing his own complete English translation of the Iliad in the hexameter style of Homer![45]

But, apart from inversions, in what way did Keats' style differ even in his iambic pentameter poetry that, in 1820, carried his outstanding ode *To Autumn*? This is the poem that 30 years ago Reeves described as being of 'resignation' while containing, in the images of Autumn evidence for the use of all the body's senses; sight, touch, smell, taste, and hearing.[46] In my opinion, with my cardiological background, at his best Keats used long a's, e's, o's, and s's, etc., which cloaks his iambic metre and allows a flow of language that first mimics then enhances the reader's pulse beat as the heart rhythm varies with phases of respiration; a condition known to clinicians as sinus arrhythmia. Add, to this rhythm and phrasing, Keats' imagination and imagery and there you have the difference especially when his syllables are not spent on the metre but the cadence rolls the metre on.

Lockhart's tachycardia of resentment would ensure he missed the rhythm of Keats' verse. His aggressive, competitive, and attacking behaviour could aggravate his raised heart beat. Such a destructive adrenaline surge of irrational criticism was, of course, not new. It has been a common theme throughout history. Unfortunately even today intelligent but inadequate people in various domains cannot look beyond their envy about the excellence of others[47,48] — but as we turn to Keats' heavily criticised *Endymion* we read:

> But this is human life: the war, the deeds,
> The disappointment, the anxiety,
> Imagination's struggles, far and nigh, All human;
> bearing in themselves this good,
> That they are still the air, the subtle food,
> To make us feel existence, and to show
> How quiet death is.[49]

Is this an example of Keats' *Negative Capability*[50] which allowed him to be '... capable of being in uncertainties, mysteries, doubts, without any irritable reaching after fact and reason....'?[51] Perhaps—but there is much in his poetry that is morose and given the background of the accidental death of his father when Keats was nine; his mother dying six years later (from presumed tuberculosis); and then his brother, Tom, coughing tuberculous blood in 1818 and dead within a year, should we be surprised? Indeed, what Keats had seen on the wards during his work as a surgical dresser, as well as his well documented unhappiness with surgery in those days before anaesthesia, allows us to understand some reasons for his melancholy; let alone the biting criticism his poetry had faced. Had Keats finally realised that the Greek world he admired (as also the later Roman) was also full of jealousy?[52] Was Keats' account of *Negative Capability* an explanation of his escape from reality? Has this concept been inadequately dealt with by previous writers because they were non-medical and even by Walter Jackson Bate,[53] who gave this subject a lifetime study? Despite his medical expertise did Osler, in his lecture on Keats: the apothecary poet, at Johns Hopkins in 1896,[54] become lost in his own definition that 'The poet is a "light and winged and holy thing", whose inspiration, genius, faculty, whatever we may choose to call it, is allied to madness—he is possessed or inspired' ... and as a result of this higher flight of reasoning, did Osler overlook what could well be the key matter? I have already mentioned the care-less freedoms that echo in Keats' poetry. Are the experiences away from reality shown in his imagery in his ode *To a*

15

Nightingale, the dream in *The Fall of Hyperion,* and the ballad *La Belle Dame sans Merci* due to his use of botanical drugs? Moreover, does Keats' awareness and contentment in drug-induced indolence add to the story?[55]

Some have speculated that there are other explanations for Keats' illness and possibly even his death. In 1817 he described using mercury.[56] This has led several to suggest that Keats had contracted what was then life-threatening syphilis; despite the fact that mercury was used as a remedy for other ills (for example, in 1819 Walter Scott was taking mercury for 'gall-stone colic').[57] Further, as I have already written, Keats had much to be depressed about. But biographical Chinese whispers and repetition have assisted unproven allegations that Keats was infected with syphilis. This allows us to recall lines from Lewis Carroll's poem, The Hunting of the Snark, '... what I tell you three times is true'.[58] This lie has been applied to Keats; John Hunter, the father of British surgery;[59] and Randolph Churchill whose doctor, Thomas Buzzard, became widely known to diagnose syphilis without his patients having real evidence of it.[60] Perhaps this is not surprising since it is a phenomenon occurring in those afraid they may contract venereal disease; and also may be used as a stigmatising slander in attempts to destroy a reputation by repetition, showing spite similar to that Lockhart repeatedly poured out against Keats. Indeed, as Harold Nicolson so succinctly stated 50 years ago, 'There are few things more vulgar ...

than the intellectuals' jealousy of a genius'.[61]

Considering these offensive speculations about Keats, after intensive investigation in 1925, Lowell concluded, '... although it is possible that Keats did contract syphilis, there is no proof whatsoever that he did, since his symptoms, so far as we can tell, are perfectly attributable to tuberculosis alone.'[62] As Somerset Maugham stated 30 years ago, 'The faculty for myth is innate in the human race. It seizes with avidity upon any incidents, surprising or mysterious, in the career of those who have distinguished themselves from their fellows, and invents a legend to which it then attaches a fanatical belief. ... The incidents of the legend become the hero's surest passport to immortality.'[63]

While Keats had been happy with indolence, living suddenly became a matter of urgency. His sense of *Negative Capability* first described in his letter to his brothers in December 1817 had, by April 1819, a reason to fade. He had met and was falling in love with Fanny Brawne.

But matters changed more dramatically and irreversibly when, by candlelight one February night in 1820, he saw a spot of blood on his pillow and recognised the implications. One hundred years after Keats' death such a pilot haemoptysis was described by Sir Thomas Horder as a diagnostic sign of tuberculosis in young men.[64]

Keats' health deteriorated. The fresh air of Rome

and help from a Dr Clark offered the only hopes of survival. So, parting from Fanny Brawne, he set off with the artist Joseph Severn[65] as his companion.

After leaving England the violence of the Scottish attacks on Keats' poetry continued. Matters became so hot that one of his defenders was killed in a duel after his challenge to Lockhart was shifted to another.[66] The rest of Keats' story is well known and I will only touch upon it here. After a delay because of his ship's quarantine, Keats entered Naples on 31st October 1820, his 25th birthday, then travelled to Rome for what he hoped would be a rapid convalescence. But 100 days later he died.

Joseph Severn had nursed Keats in Rome daily and attentively. His letters to Keats' friends well describe Keats' final days. For our purposes they can be summarised by referring to Severn's letter dated the 25th and 26th January 1821[67] when he stated, '… poor Keats is now upon his death bed— he has shown worse symptoms every day—clay-like expectoration—in large quantities—night sweats—ghastly wasting-away of his body and extremities….' And, Severn continues, '…I pray God speedily to lift him up—his suffering now is beyond description…. The hardest point between [us] is that cursed [unused] bottle of Opium [Keats had purchased this some time before they sailed] — he had determined on taking this the instant his recovery should stop—he says … and but for me [Severn kept the opium from him and would not let Keats take it] —he would have swallowed this draught 3 Months since—in the ship—he says 3 wretched months I have kept him alive…. Keats is desiring his death with dreadfull [sic] earnestness….'

Some two years previously Keats had written to his brother and sister-in-law: 'Do you not see how necessary a World of Pains and troubles is to school Intelligence and make it a Soul? A Place where the heart must feel and suffer in a thousand diverse ways.'[68] Brave words when he was well but as daily he lay enduring what he described as 'this posthumous life of mine',[69] his dying was an unnecessarily hard travail. The opium that Severn and Clark denied him could have helped to ease his passage, as could the cough-suppressing and narcotic actions of other botanicals about which Keats knew—such as hemlock, datura, and henbane—but none were administered.

On the day following his death, Dr Clark and Dr Luby with an Italian Surgeon opened Keats' body and found that the lungs were 'intirely [sic] destroyed' and 'the cells were quite gone'[70] hence the use of the word *consumption* in those days.[71]

I do not think there is any rational person who would wish to endure such prolonged and distressful dying as did John Keats[72] and especially when appropriate palliation was available.

So what is euthanasia and is there a case for it? Euthanasia literally means achieving a good, comfortable, death. Something I am sure we would all wish for ourselves at the appropriate time. To this writer it does not mean enforced or legalised killing.

Unfortunately today, the term 'euthanasia' has been hi-jacked. It now commonly means that when a person has unrelieved symptoms a doctor will induce death with a lethal injection or draught.

Perhaps we have forgotten the historical background to the medical murders committed for social engineering or eugenic reasons and that these started from small beginnings. As Dowbiggin[73] has pointed out, the Nazi-era of euthanasia, with the murder of millions, was not an accident of history but a policy with a powerful ancestry dating back to the late nineteenth century. The contrasting message is as clear. Indeed, those who doubt that it is and are still wishing to pursue the legalising of euthanasia for the relief of physical and emotional distress, should know that when civil libertarians cried out in America for euthanasia to be legalised, Professor Kamisar, the Minnesota law professor, warned that the 'legal machinery initially designed to kill those who are a nuisance to themselves may someday engulf those who are a nuisance to others'. Furthermore, seeking or offering to induce death with a lethal injection when a person has unrelieved symptoms overlooks the important and simple question: why are the symptoms unrelieved?
Repeated failure to answer this question is closely

tied to perceptions about and the practical realities concerning the present poor quality of what is euphemistically called 'the end-of-life' while forgetting that the end of life is death, about which nothing corrective can be done. Therefore, the term we should use is not 'the end of life' but by placing the word 'care' first, draw attention to where humanity should be, namely: providing 'care at the ending of life', or more simply the old phrase 'care for the dying'. At this stage one of the problems at the bedside can be that clinical professionals are at a loss about what to do, and their ability to turn a 'blind eye' to the problems provides, for them, an easy evading answer. This curious paradox of illness behaviour is the result of at least three factors: firstly, the virtual absence today of those life-threatening epidemic diseases that previously provided almost daily experience with dying patients of all ages; secondly, the easy availability of persistent diagnostic and therapeutic endeavour associated with high-technology medicine amongst which to hide one's ignorance about effective palliative care; and also, the failure to pause at the bedside and listen and respond to patients as they describe their anxieties and needs. One of the key answers here lies in effective updating education of both under- and clinical post-graduates with universities, collegiate bodies, and also National Health Service Trusts accepting and monitoring their responsibilities. All bedside professionals must have at least a basic knowledge about palliative care. This can then be used to impart a confidence to dying patients, their relatives, and friends as well as to fellow student professionals, especially when more specialist help is readily available as required. All of this can relieve immediate anxieties, promote effective care, and lessen the panics about dying that invariably heighten the cry for legalised euthanasia.

When last year Joan Bakewell, the appointed 'old peoples' Tsar', was reported as saying that 'The elderly should *not* be kept alive indefinitely by technology ... when their identity has ceased to exist'[74] – with certain safeguards we may agree. But when a terminally-ill 13-years-old girl, who had been treated for leukaemia, was widely reported in the national press as having to go to the Law Court, to defend and win her right *not* to have a heart transplant forced upon her by a hospital; when a woman, aged 45, had also to seek the Court's advice on whether her husband would face prosecution if he assisted her to travel abroad to where assisted suicide is legal; when a paralysed ex-rugby player, aged 23, had already committed suicide in this way; and, when, as evidence of inadequacies in clinical care, millions of pounds of compensation are still being paid by the National Health Service for negligence – we should not be surprised if questions are asked as to whether the clinical and social care of the living *and* the dying are being managed properly in this country? If not, why not? Or, again, if it is pointed out that 35 years ago a medical student stated, 'We come to clinical medicine with humanity and after three years they have educated it out of us',[75] is it reasonable to suggest that this is why things have not changed? Is it *as* reasonable to ask: do the medical schools and Royal Colleges lag far behind in ensuring there are adequate standards of personal medical care at the bedside; has the General Medical Council, with its publicly stated ethos of 'ensuring good medical practice', been silent about this matter for too long; and, does Bristol have the only university giving a strong lead on 'medical humanities' that will be carried to the bedside?[76]

Around 500,000 people die in England each year. The Department of Health's commitment to provide £12m in funding for the End of Life Care Programme from 2004 to 2007[77] may, in 2009, still be ongoing. Regretfully, there is no avoiding the fact that while the National Health Service delivers 380 million treatments it receives more than 135,000 complaints a year. The Healthcare Commission only reviews 9,000 of these.[78] It is a matter of concern that in April 2009 the Healthcare Commission was disbanded and its successor, the Care Quality Commission, will not take on its complaints handling role. Instead, these will be dealt with by the Trusts themselves and, if complainants are still unhappy, the Health Service Ombudsman. Such changes have abolished the independent review stage carried out by the Healthcare Commission. While it has been stated that 'only a very small fraction of the total treatments led to complaints', these involved more than 135,000 patients and as many families each year. It is not just the quantity of complaints but their quality that matters [as Shipman[79] and Allitt[80] showed], especially when Trusts will 'sit as judge and jury on their own failings'.[81] In 2008 a widely cited Healthcare Commission's Press Release said '54% of complaints about acute hospitals related to care surrounding death'.[82] This is an emotionally charged period for any family and this large percentage highlights the feelings of relatives over failures in the standards of care.[83]

There is little doubt that cancer leading to the end of life can be well managed by the Hospice movement and Macmillan nurses. But more patients are dying from heart failure than all forms of cancer and current national strong feeling is about recognising and managing these needs—as well as the needs of people of all ages who have non-cancer but similarly protracted conditions.

There are too many instances of family members, still struggling to accept their impending loss, refusing to accept the explanations offered by doctors. Here, obviously, inadequate time and thought has been given by key-players, including the medical professionals.

I have great difficulty in *not* believing that this failure is related to the need for the shortest possible duration of 'finished consultant episodes'; the achievement of five-star ratings; and performance related targets. There are parallel complaints about poor standards of hygiene, nursing care, and bad staff attitudes, unacceptable at any time but particularly upsetting for those grieving. There is also a disturbing number of cases where truth has been hidden and caring families have received misleading or contradictory information from those in charge of their relative and here I will not use the word 'caring'.[84]

All of this adds to heightened national concern that fosters demands that to accelerate the end of life 'assisted suicide' be legalised.

Amid this ferment what may be forgotten is, as Koenig has stated, 'The request for assisted suicide is often a cry for help, a cry of fear, a cry of desperation. Rather than support and assist the patient in ending their life, physicians must identify those factors that underlie the suffering (psychological and physical) and do everything they can to relieve them.'[85] And there too I stand firmly because we should be into care not killing.

Is it only a cynic who thinks that the National Health Service has developed a "command and control" structure that is too far removed from the immediacy of patient care. With equally bureaucratic attempts at public relations do busy providers find themselves more concerned with service costs rather than patients' needs? For example, can one ask how many Trusts now have effective, dedicated Dignity Champions to facilitate local education other than the twenty-three showing excellence who were visited for the 2007 report on Caring for Dignity.[86] What are the relevant principles for the care of the dying that are being used? The commonly used Liverpool Care Pathway for the dying[87] is only appropriate after an accurate diagnosis of the patient's clinical condition has been made and every reversible condition treated, even if subsequently that treatment is withdrawn.[88]

So what other principles need to be considered if dying is to be a humane experience for us all? More importantly, perhaps, with what authority do I speak on these matters?

My practical experience as a physician includes listening to and sharing the emotional and other needs of hundreds of dying patients for almost 50 years; and the concerns of their relatives, as well as medical and para-clinical staff – while producing peer-reviewed work about the management of dying.

I know that the high emotions of distressed relatives around the deathbed can be at least partially if not completely assuaged once time is taken to listen and answer all their questions. For some, particularly after the Shipman case, a greater time may be required to state that potent analgesics and sedatives do *not* mean that death is deliberately accelerated – although as part of palliative treatment it may not be postponed.[89] Equally it is important to point out tactfully to relatives who – with their own emotional needs, may have developed the 'you-won't-let-mum-die-will-you-doctor?' position, and request inappropriate resuscitation attempts — that the dying person should not be made to practise how to die before they are finally allowed to do so. This phrase is also especially relevant to those clinical practitioners of the 'not-allowed-to-die-syndrome' variety, who do not know when to stop treatment and investigation and have not even considered the question 'Are you, doctor/nurse, doing this for the patient or is the patient doing it for you?'[90] This is one of the reasons for some people being afraid of dying. They want a rapid enforced exit because they believe their symptoms may *not* be controlled while their life is artificially prolonged in a body that is merely existing and still feeling pain and distress; hence the cries for legislation to allow active killing.

I have little doubt that until there is a widespread change in clinical practice the diagnosis so often overlooked or evaded will continue to be that the patient is dying. Furthermore, apprehensions about clinical care and requests for euthanasia will continue while courtesy, communication, common sense, and adequate clinical ability do not attend at the bedside and when on ward rounds, or in the home, medical practitioners of all grades pass by without discussing matters with the patient face-to-face and with the relatives as well. Roger Henderson QC hit the nail firmly on the head in his Inner Temple Ormrod Lecture[91] last year when he discussed the decline of the quality of professionalism in both Medicine and the Law. He pointed out that their service to the public needs to be restored and not the least because 'We are all actual or potential patients....' This view was echoed in a Royal College Journal in December 2008 which described the centrality of the doctor-patient relationship and overall aims for service improvements.[92] Neither of the writers produced specific *objectives* that would lead to direct mechanisms for change; but this task requires more than a sentence or two.

A patient approaching the end of life today can be like John Keats, who, although attended constantly by a caring friend and visited daily by a doctor, had no relief from his distressing symptoms despite effective herbal remedies which were available and could have ensured his freedom from suffering. It is still surprising today that the 'care of the dying' can be so inadequate. In 2009, we should begin to recognise the need to protect patients from a "Keatsian experience". Are not the principles of palliation for those dying not only well described but readily accessible in textbooks? Do we really need to recall the questions posed almost 30 years ago by Professor Williamson, 'What would I wish if the patient were my own Mother?, or, even more pertinently: What if I were the patient?'[93]

As far as John Keats and we are concerned, do matters stop here?

Nine days before he died, on the 23rd February 1821, Keats requested that his gravestone should bear the simple words, 'Here lies one whose name is writ in water'.[94]

Some have imagined that he was the first to use this phrase but in a Jacobean play written in 1610 entitled Philaster: or, Love Lies a Bleeding,[95] there is:

Your memory shall be as soul behind you
As you are living, all your better deeds
Shall be in water writ ...[96]

Keats was an ardent fan of Shakespeare who in the first folio edition of his play King Henry VIII wrote:

Men's evil manners live in brass:
their virtues we write in water.[97]

Could that be Keats' meaning?

Some time ago, while researching Keats' interest in painting and sculpture, I found in an anonymous preface to a book published in 1658, almost 50 years after Shakespeare's Henry VIII, concerning the Art of painting in water colours, the statement:

Your fame shall (spite of proverbs) make it plain
To write in water's not to write in vain — [98]

Eighty years after Keats' death, Rudyard Kipling, a future Nobel Prize Winner for Literature, noted for the fluency of his ideas and ability to capture the moment of inspiration, and also known for his belief that *all* his writing was done at the command of a personal Daemon,[99] wrote a short story entitled *Wireless* that '…was generated by his excitement of finding — in the new development of wireless telegraphy — parallels to his conception of the mysterious nature of inspiration.'[100]

This story was about a consumptive poet and referred to:

a girl-friend Fanny,
Apothecaries Hall,
coughing and haemoptysis,
arterial blood,
a collection of letters,
the rack,
Keats' poems,
a rich port-wine coloured mixture frothing at the top,
St Agnes' Eve,
Keats himself,
transient unconsciousness with swiftly dilated pupils, and,
death before the year was out.

This account demonstrates Kipling's familiarity with the life and works of John Keats.[101] Why should he not use Keats when 'botany had long been one of Kipling's hobbies and old English herbals his delight'.[102]

Further, it is known that Kipling needed to borrow a rhythm, from a hymn tune or somewhere else, to help him compose his verses.[103] His borrowings from the works of others are amusingly described in his poem entitled *When Omer smote his blooming lyre*. As Fischer echoed a few years ago, '...all writing involves borrowing and adaptation, not "creation"....'[104]

But life is full of surprises, as Professor Heinrich, Professor of Pharmacognosy, found when he discovered the plant known as Atropa belladonna - Deadly Nightshade growing just *outside* the London School of Pharmacy.[105]

Just as Keats had diagnosed his own tuberculosis and ultimate death from the sudden solitary spot of blood he coughed onto his pillow, so Kipling's use of the word 'rack' in his *Wireless* leads us to one particular letter Keats had written to Fanny Brawne.[106] In this letter Keats adds, in the jealousy of his distress, and for the first and only time in his known works: 'You must be mine to die upon the rack if I want you....'

... and in a few lines before this demand there is a particular rhythm where Keats wrote:

If you could really what is call'd enjoy yourself ...
If you can smile in peoples' faces,
and wish them to admire you now, ...

Are these few lines among Keats' writings where the inspiring daemon offered a rhythm for Kipling's poem 'IF'?

The way to cope with malevolent social challenges, slanders, and difficulties that were faced by Keats in his short life, and have to be faced by others in theirs today, is found in almost every line of 'IF'. Was Kipling inspired to write 'IF' with Keats in mind after writing *Wireless*, which drew so richly on Keats' life, his poetry, illness, and death?

Although some have said 'IF' was written for Dr Leander Starr Jameson there are good reasons for thinking this untrue. Jameson led about 600 of his countrymen in such a shambles of a raid against the Boers in southern Africa, that the 'Jameson Raid'[107] is considered a major factor in starting the Boer War four years later. A war subsequently described by Kipling as 'a war of fools'.[108]

Fifteen years after the Jameson debacle, and nearly 100 years ago this year, Kipling's 'IF' first appeared with his collection of stories entitled *Rewards and Fairies*.[109] In this book two of the tales[110] were inspired by historically-based promptings from a physician distantly related to Kipling; who, like Keats, had experienced prolonged, severe, and demoralising criticism from the press. Like Keats, this man died in physical distress from a chest infection, carrying to his grave wounds of rejection by colleagues.[111] Kipling sent him a first copy of *Rewards and Fairies* which contains amongst its theme of healing the relevant and strengthening words of 'IF' from which this physician would have benefited considerably. — But who was he and why was 'IF' so important to him?[112]

His name? ... William Osler.

Of the very many works the then challenged Osler published and the quotations attributed to him, the most relevant and I think the best to encourage us to work with understanding, sympathy, and compassion while caring for the dying is one that has 2000 years' authority behind it, namely: 'To serve the art of medicine as it should be served, one must love his fellow-men.'[113]

Notes

1   Keats J. On first looking into Chapman's Homer. *John Keats's Poems.* [ed.] Gerald Bullet. Dent: London. Everyman's Library. 1969. p.35. [Keats' uses the word 'demesne' (a Sovereign's territory) at the end of line six. This is the Anglo-French spelling of the Old French word 'demeine' pronounced 'de-meen' and rhyming with the line endings 'seen', 'been', and 'serene'.]

2   'Well, then, we were put in possession of the Homer of Chapman, and to work we went, turning to some of the 'famousest' passages, as we had scrappily known them in Pope's version. ... Chapman supplied us with many an after-feast; but it was in the teeming wonderment of this, his first introduction, that, when I came down to breakfast the next morning, I found upon my table a letter with no other inclosure [*sic*] than his famous sonnet, 'On first looking into Chapman's Homer.' We had

parted, as I have already said, at day-spring; yet he contrived that I should receive the poem, from a distance of nearly two miles, before 10, A.M.' [Clarke C. Cowden Clarke on Keats. [in] Matthews GM [editor]. *Keats: the critical heritage*. London. Routledge & Kegan Paul. 1971. pp.390-391.]

3   The full sense of this sonnet can be captured by using many of the stresses suggested by Johnson and, in this writer's opinion, others should be added to capture the full sense of Keats' imagery. [Johnson AL. Formal Messages in Keats's Sonnets. *DQR Studies in Literature, The Challenge of Keats: Bicentenary Essays 1795-1995*, edited by A. Christensen, L. Jones, G. Galigani and A. Johnson. 2000;28:95-111 (17).]

4   It was not Cortez who discovered the Pacific but Balboa. The three syllables of 'Bal-bo-a' do not fit the line; whereas 'Cort-ez' keeps the balance right.

5   Johnson overstates his case about anagrammatic inventions. Keats was a great punster. See for example his letter to Charles and Maria Dilke dated 24 January 1819. [Forman MB. [editor] *The letters of John Keats*. 1947. p.281] where Keats has written at the end 'I beg leaf to withdraw all my Puns — they are all wash, an base uns —'. The 'anagrams' in this sonnet are at the end on the octet and sestet. "Speak out" can be punned into "Keats' [s]pout"; and, "silent peak" into "li[k]en Keats" — that is, as Keats had done when he stared across the sea from the South coast cliffs at Margate in 1816 before he wrote this sonnet - with the "p" being 'silent.

6   Homer [author], George Chapman [translator]. *The Iliad and Odyssey*. London. Wordsworth Classics of the World's literature. 2002. p. xlvi.

7   Scott GF. *Joseph Severn: letters and memoirs*.

34

Aldershot. Ashgate. 2005. p.632.

8   Colvin S. *John Keats: his life and poetry: his friends,
     critics, and after-fame*. Charles Scribners's Sons. 1925.
     p.521. See also: Macbeth G. *John Gibson Lockhart: a
     critical study*. University of Illinois. 1935. p.116.
9   'Who read for me the sonnet swelling loudly / up to
     its climax, and then dying proudly?' [in] Keats J.
     Letter to Mr CC Clarke. September 1816. [in] Scott
     GF. *Selected letters of John Keats*. Harvard University
     Press. 2002. p.5.
10   Lawrence TE [author], cited by Alberto Manguel [in]
     Homer's The Iliad and the Odyssey: a biography.
     London. Atlantic Books. 2007. p.32.
11   Payne R. *The gold of Troy: the story of the archaeologist,
     Heinrich Schliemann*. Reader's Digest Condensed
     Books. 1978. p.256.
12   Manguel. op.cit. p.57.
13   Pope A [author], Simeon Underwood [writer].
     *English translators of Homer: from George Chapman to
     Christopher Logue. Writers and their work*. Northcote
     House Publishers Ltd. 1998. p.35. It is noted in
     passing that Pope's translation became so popular
     that he made a profit of £10,000 from his Homer
     translation; see: Alexander Pope [author], Pat
     Rogers [editor]. *Alexander Pope* (The Oxford Poetry
     Library). OUP. 1994. p.x.
14   Chambers R. [ed.]. *The Book of Days*. London: W & R
     Chambers. 1832;2:511. 'From school he [Keats] was
     taken, at the age of fifteen, and apprenticed for five
     years to a surgeon and apothecary at Edmonton; an
     easy distance from Enfield, so that he used to walk
     over whenever he liked to see the Clarkes and
     borrow books. He [Keats] was an insatiable and
     indiscriminate reader, and shewed [*sic*] no peculiar
     bias in his tastes, until, in 1812, he obtained in loan

Spenser's *Fairy Queen*. That poem lit the fire of his
genius. He could now speak of nothing but Spenser.
A world of delight seemed revealed to him. 'He
ramped through the scenes of the romance,' writes
Mr Clarke 'like a young horse turned into a spring
meadow;' ' he got whole passages by heart, which
he would repeat to any listener; and would dwell
with ecstasy on fine phrases, such as that of 'the sea-
shouldering whale.' This intense enjoyment soon led
to his trying his own hand at verse, and the chief
end of his existence became henceforward the
reading and writing of poetry. With his friend
Cowden Clarke, then a youth like himself, he spent
long evenings in enthusiastic discussion of the
English poets, shewing a characteristic preference
for passages of sweet sensuous description, such as
are found in the minor poems of Chaucer,
Shakspeare, [*sic*] and Milton, and throughout
Spenser, rather than for those dealing with the
passions of the human heart. By Clarke he was
introduced to Greek poetry, through the medium of
translations. They commenced Chapman's *Homer*
one evening, and read till daylight, Keats sometimes
shouting aloud with delight as some passage of
special energy struck his imagination. Therewith
began that remarkable affiliation of his mind to the
Greek mythology, which gave to his work so
marked a form and colour.'

15   de Almeida H. *Romantic Medicine and John Keats*.
OUP. Oxford. 1991. p.169. 'Alexander Marcet was an
authority on urinary calculi. … He gave the earliest
description of alkaptonuria.' His work, on the
chemical composition of urine and calculi, helped
lay the foundations for our present knowledge.' See:
Rosenfeld L. The chemical work of Alexander and

Jane Marcet. *Clinical Chemistry* 2001; 47:784–792;
Coley NG. Alexander Marcet (1770-1822), physician
and animal chemist. *Medical History* 1968; 12:394-
402; and, Knight D. Communicating chemistry: the
frontier between popular books and textbooks in
Britain during the first half of the nineteenth
century. [in] *Communicating chemistry: textbooks and
their audiences, 1789-1939.* [eds.] Anders Lundgren
and Bernadette Bensaude-Vincent. European studies
in science history and the arts, Vol. 3. Science
History Publications, USA: A Division of Watson
Publishing International: Canton, MA, 2000. pp.187-
205.

16   http://en.wikipedia.org/wiki/Datura_stramonium.

17   Barton R. Who ever heard of Doctor Keats? *New
York State Journal of Medicine* 1977;77(2):244-246. This
states on p.244 : 'A statute of July 12, 1815, was
pushed by G. M. Burrows, M.D. (St. Andrews) 1771-
1846, England's Simon Flexner, who kept a private
asylum at Clapham. It enacted that no person
should practice as an apothecary in any part of
England or Wales unless he had been examined by a
court of examiners and received wherefrom a
certificate. From August 1, 1815, to be admitted to
the examination, a candidate had to have served five
years' apprenticeship and at least six months of
hospital training.'

18   de Almeida. ibid. p.87.

19   Rollins HE. *The Keats Circle: letters and papers, 1816-
1878.* Harvard University Press. 1948; 1:267. 'One
Morning early in February (before his death) I
[Joseph Severn] was delighted to find the Spring
had commenced here – and when the poor fellow
[Keats] awoke I told him of it – I told him I had seen
some trees in blossom – this had a most dreadful

effect on him – I had mistaken the point – he shed
tears most bitterly – and said – "The spring was
always inchantment [*sic*] to me – I could get away
from suffering in watching the growth of a little
flower – it was real delight to me – it was part of my
very soul – perhaps the only happiness I have had
in the world – has been the silent growth of Flowers
– Ah! Why did you let me know this – why show
me that this comfort is gone – that I shall never see
the Spring again – I hoped to die before the spring
came – O I would to God – that I were in my grave –
quiet and insensible to these ghastly hands – these
knobbed knees [*sic*] – The grave – with Flowers on its
top – send me to it now" ....'

20   Lethe was the supposed river of Hades whose
     waters when drunk caused forgetfulness.
21   In Greek mythology, Hippocrene was the name of a
     fountain on Mount Helicon. It was sacred to the
     Muses and stated to have been formed by the
     hooves of Pegasus. Its name literally translates to
     'Horse's Fountain'.
22   The syllabic flow of this and the associated lines
     have a cadence reminiscent of that in Dylan
     Thomas' *Under Milk Wood*.
23   'St John's wort: if you pinch the leaves or the petals
     they give out reddish purple stain—the "blood of St.
     John". There are many ancient superstitions
     regarding this herb. Its name *hypericum* is derived
     from the Greek that means 'over an apparition', a
     reference to the belief that the herb was so
     obnoxious to evil spirits that a whiff of it would
     cause them to fly. Keeping this herb in your garden
     was believed to protect you from fairy trickery.
     Carrying a few stems of the foliage was an old way
     to avoid being 'fairy-led', or lost and confused while

wandering through the local enchanted forest.' See: http://www.anniesremedy.com/herb_detail147.php

24 Sullivan J. A note on the death of Socrates. *The Classical Quarterly, New Series* 2001;51(2);608-610.

25 Jowett B [translator]. *Dialogues of Plato.* Pocket Books Inc. 1957. p.159.

26 Hibbert C. *George IV: Regent and King, 1811-1830.* Readers Union. 1975. p.14. 'According to Princess Charlotte he [George IV] was also taking "a great quantity" of hemlock which was now his only means of getting any sleep.'

27 *The Daily Telegraph.* 'Hemlock' coma of top brain surgeon. 23 October 2001.

28 Such confusion between hemlock and parsley or celery was described in 1816. See: Salisbury W. *The botanist's companion, or an introduction to the knowledge of practical botany, and the uses of plants: either growing wild in Great Britain, or cultivated for the purposes of agriculture, medicine, rural oeconomy, or the arts* 1816;2:141.

29 Slowing of the pulse is one of the depressant effects of opium and an agonist effect of hemlock.

30 One of the effects of opium.

31 Another of the effects of opium.

32 Lloyd M. Keats's embodied: The Tempest, synaesthesia and contemporary brain science. *The Keats-Shelley Review* 2008;22:101.

33 Silenus was alleged to be a companion and tutor to the wine god Dionysus and was regarded as a notorious consumer of wine, he was usually drunk. When intoxicated, he was said to possess special knowledge and the power of prophecy.

34 Colvin. op.cit. p.379.

35 Laudanum was the commonplace tranquilliser and painkiller of the day. See: Powell N. *George Crabbe:*

     an English life (1754-1832) Pimlico. 2004. p.125.

36   Hayter A. *Opium and the romantic imagination.* Faber and Faber. London. 1968. p.311.

37   Rollins. op cit. pp. 245-247. Here Lockhart's attack was described as 'violent, cruel, and ungentle-manly'; and see also Colvin. op.cit. pp.306-307. The phrases used by Lockhart given above are the usual ones repeated in various textbooks. For a more complete appreciation of the continuing and at times the unseemly, if not vitriolic, comments of Lockhart and others see: Matthews op.cit. pp.19-26.

38   Macbeth 1935. op.cit. p.32.

39   ibid. p.115.

40   [Author not available.] Lockhart, John Gibson. *The Columbia Encyclopedia.* Sixth Edition. 2008.

41   Dr. Sangra'do of Vall'adolid'. Entry taken from: the *Dictionary of phrase and fable*, edited by the Rev. E. Cobham Brewer, LL.D. and revised in 1895. The actions of Dr. Sangrado [spelling as used by Lockhart] were referred to by Henry Fielding in his then popular book *Joseph Andrews*, 1792.

42   Marsh GL. *Keats and the periodicals of his time.* Modern Philology 1934;32:37-53.

43   Daiches D. *Robert Fergusson.* Scottish Academic Press. 1982. p.11. The hurt of national pride remained after the 1707 Act of Union; when '...English was firmly established as the language of published prose discourse in Scotland, the language to be learned in school as the accepted mode of utterance, and as the language of those poets who sought an English audience....'

44   In 1835, Lockhart published *The works of Robert Burns together with an account of his life*. There are various editions of this work with corrections following its original 1828 publication in Edinburgh.

45 Macbeth, op.cit. p.50. 'The metre of a poem is its pulse beat or metron. The hexameter has six metrons (feet) of dactyls (fingers). Each dactyl has a long first syllable followed by two short;...' [e.g. High in the | sky is the | star to see; | call-ing you | home to be | near to me.]

46 Reeves J. *Understanding poetry*. Pan Books Ltd. 1978. pp.181-182.

47 Mouly S, Sankaran J. The tall poppy syndrome in New Zealand: an exploratory investigation. [in] Transcending boundaries: integrating people, processes and systems. *Proceedings of the 2nd Annual Conference of the International Association of Insight and Action*, Brisbane, Australia, September 2000; pp.264-268.

48 Mouly S, Sankaran J. The enactment of envy within organizations: insights from a New Zealand academic department. *Journal of applied behavioral science* 2002;38(1);36-56. [Some 80 years previously, however, Hearn described this behaviour as, 'The difficult people to deal with are those who attract us by an apparent refinement and gentleness and kind ness — though secretly watching for an opportunity to do us all possible injury.' See: Hearn L [author]. *A history of English literature* (1907). R Tanabe, T Ochiai, and I Nishizaki [editors]. The Hokuseido Press. Tokyo. Revised edition, 1970. pp.676-677.]

49 Keats J. Endymion, Book II, lines 153-159. *The poetical works of John Keats*. [ed.] HW Garrod. London. OUP. 1956. p.83.

50 This has been described as 'creative passiveness'. See: Hardy B. Keats, Coleridge and negative capability. *Notes and queries* 5 July 1952; pp.299-301. 'Negative capability' should not be confused with Keats' observation that '... the simple imaginative

Mind may have its rewards in the repeti(ti)on of its own silent Working coming continually on the Spirit with a fine Suddenness — ....' Forman. op. cit. p.68.

51   Forman. ibid. p.72. [Whereas, Coleridge described 'the capability of being stimulated into sensation' in his Letter to John Thelwall, 31 December 1796. See: Coleridge ST [author] HJ Jackson [editor] *The Oxford Authors: Samuel Taylor Coleridge*. OUP. 1985. p.492.]

52   Livingstone RW. *The Greek genius and its meaning to us*. OUP. 1915. p.148. [In my opinion [BL] the conflicts Keats faced, in his consideration of the harsh reality of the criticism of his poetry, had difficulty meeting with his thoughts about the divine which he had embraced in his concepts of truth and beauty. His struggles with his religious sense have been well described [see: Ryan RM. in *Keats: the religious sense*. Princeton University Press. New Jersey. 1976] To more fully appreciate Keats' difficulties readers may be interested to read Auerbach's analysis of the legendary historic view of the works of Homer seen against the 'lived experience' of Biblical history. [See: Auerbach E. *Mimesis: the representation of reality in Western literature*. Translated by Edward W. Said. Princeton University Press. Princeton and Oxford. 2003; and also, Steiner G. Grave jubilation. *Times Literary Supplement*. 19 September 2003. pp.3-5.] Certainly, in Keats' struggles to work out the meaning of life and death for himself, it is not obvious that he was helped by reading Jeremy Taylor's two volumes entitled *Holy living and holy dying* which with much difficulty Dr Clarke found for him in Rome. Taylor had been regarded as a theologian of the first rank and his volumes, first published in 1650 and 1651, had an accepted tradition. [The modern version of

both volumes consulted by this writer was 'Taylor J. *Holy Living and Holy Dying*. Edited and annotated P. G. Stanwood. Oxford University Press, 1989.'] Although Taylor's text may appear ponderous to the average reader it has run to many editions over the centuries. Taylor's doctrine of toleration may have helped Keats but his [Keats'] statement that Lockhart should be ruined [see the main text] left Keats little room for manoeuvre as he continued for months without palliation of his symptoms while suffering and struggling to die.]]

53   See: Bate WJ. *The Sympathetic Imagination in Eighteenth-Century English criticism* ELH [English Literary History] 1945;12(2);144-164; and, Bate WJ. *John Keats*. The Belknap Press of Harvard University Press. 1963. pp.233-263; and also: Bate WJ [author]. Negative capability. [ed.] Walter Jackson Bate. *Keats: a collection of critical essays*. Prentice-Hall, Inc., New Jersey. 1964. pp.51-68. [This last text contains deletions from Bate's original text published as 'Negative Capability' [in] *John Keats* (Harvard University Press. Cambridge, Mass. 1963 compared with that held in copyright by the President and Fellows of Harvard College. See also: Bate WJ. Negative capability. [in] *Modern critical views: John Keats*. Edited with introduction by Harold Bloom. Chelsea House Publishers. New York. 1985. pp.13-28. — but this does not add anything substantial to Bate's views. The reader may also be interested to see: Forman. op.cit. 1947. p.72; and, also for example: Osler Sir W. John Keats, the apothecary poet. [in] *An Alabama student and other biographical essays*. OUP. 1908. It is interesting, as has been stated elsewhere that 'Even Keats was unable to offer a prescription to help us become poets, and we cannot

find in his letters the answer to the all-important question how to acquire 'negative capability'. [stated in: Leavy SA. John Keats's psychology of creative imagination. *The Psychoanalytic Quarterly* 1970; 39:173-197: see p.187.] It is noted that not one of these writers considered the effects of botanical drugs on Keats' passive imagination and thinking.

54 Osler op.cit. p.38.
55 On 19 March 1819, Keats wrote to his brother George and sister-in-law Georgiana. In this letter, Keats described his indolence: 'This is the only happiness; and is a rare instance of advantage in the body overpowering the Mind.' See for example the explanation in the text given to verse 2 in Keats' *Ode to indolence*: 'Ripe was the drowsy hour; The blissful cloud of summer-indolence benumb'd my eyes; my pulse grew less and less; pain had no sting, and pleasure's wreath no flower.'
56 John Keats' letter to Benjamin Bailey, 8 October 1817.
57 MacNalty (Sir) AS. *Sir Walter Scott: the wounded falcon*. London. Johnson. 1969. p.152; which describes Scott taking 'a drastic course of calomel' to relieve his attack of 'gall-stone colic'.
58 Carroll L. [Author] The Hunting of the Snark; edited by Martin Gardener as *The Annotated Snark*. Penguin. 1967. p.46.
59 Livesley B. Lecture entitled 'John Hunter's experiment' delivered at the Royal College of Surgeons of Edinburgh on 16th April 2008.
60 Reviews. *Journal of Mental Science* 1874;20:288. See also: Buzzard T. *Clinical aspects of syphilitic nervous affections*. London. J & A Churchill. 1874. p.11. 'I have little hesitation in stating my conviction [based on no evidence] that, putting aside cases of injury,

hemiplegia or paraplegia occurring in a person between twenty and forty-five years of age, which is not associated with Bright's disease, not due to embolism (from disease of the cardiac valves) is, *in at least* [enhanced text] nineteen cases out of twenty, the result of syphilis.'

61 Nicolson H. [Book review] Vulgarian of genius. *The Observer*. 15 November 1959. p.22.

62 Lowell A. *John Keats*. London: Jonathan Cape, 1925; cited by Smith H. The Strange Case of Mr. Keats's Tuberculosis. *Clinical Infectious Diseases* 2004;38:991–993. [Amy Lowell was one of the first of a long line of distinguished American biographers of Keats.]

63 Maugham WS. *The moon and sixpence*. Pan Books Ltd. 1974. p.7.

64 Horder [Sir] T. *Medical notes*. Oxford Medical Publications. 1921. p.46.

65 Severn was not a particularly close friend. He appears to have been the only one of the Keats circle who was free to accompany him to Rome.

66 Scott. 2005. ibid. p.615.

67 Rollins. op.cit. Vol.1; pp.202-205.

68 Keats J. [author] MB Forman [editor] London. 1935. 2nd edition. February 14 - May 3; 1819; p.336.

69 Joseph Severn to John Taylor, 6 March 1821. [in] Scott GE. [editor] *Selected letters of John Keats: based on the texts of Hyder Edward Rollins*. London. Harvard University Press. 2002. p.511.

70 Rollins. op.cit. Vol. 1; p.225.

71 This together with the eventual rapid onset of death suggests that Keats' final exitus was due to pneumothorax. This would explain why when Keats' body was opened it was '…found that the lungs were 'intirely [*sic*] destroyed' and 'the cells were quite gone' hence the use of the word

consumption in those days.

72 After John Keats' death, Fanny Brawne wrote to his sister Fanny 'You do not, you never can know how much he has suffered. So much that I do believe, were it in my power I would not bring him back.' Brawne F. [cited by] Richardson J [in] *Fanny Brawne: a biography*. London. Thames and Hudson 1952. p.66.

73 Dowbiggin I. *A concise history of euthanasia: life, death, God, and medicine*. New York. Rowman & Littlefield Publishers Inc. 2007. pp.92 & 107.

74 Beckford M. Allow dementia sufferers to die, says old people's 'tsar' Bakewell. *The Daily Telegraph*. Monday, November 17, 2008; p.13. Subsequently archived at Telegraph.co.uk as: Don't keep pensioners alive indefinitely, says old people tsar Dame Joan Bakewell. By Martin Beckford, Social Affairs Correspondent. Last Updated: 2:56AM GMT 17 Nov 2008. See also: http://www.telegraph.co.uk/news/newstopics/debates/3467820/Dont-keep-pensioners-alive-indefinitely-says-Governments-old-people-tsar-Dame-Joan-Bakewell.html; 'But Dame Joan told The Daily Telegraph that she does not believe advancements in medicine and technology should mean the elderly are kept alive for as long as possible regardless of the quality of their lives.'

75 Gale J, Livesley B. Attitudes towards geriatrics: a report of the King's survey. *Age & Ageing* 1974;3:49-53.

76 The Intercalated BA in Medical Humanities at the University of Bristol is available to students from other medical schools.

77 Department of Health. Building on the best: choice, responsiveness and equity. 2003.

78   'NHS trusts failing patients over complaints. Almost
     half of grievances not dealt with properly, says
     Health Commission.' *Press Association and
     Guardian.co.uk.* Monday 16 February 2009 12.43
     GMT. http://www.guardian.co.uk/society/2009/
     feb/16/health-commission-nhs-complaints
79   The Shipman Inquiry published its final report on
     27 January 2005 and was decommissioned at Easter
     2005. See: http://www.the-shipman-inquiry.org.uk/
     home.asp.
80   'Serial killer nurse Allitt must serve 30 years.'
     http://www.guardian.co.uk/uk/2007/dec/06/
     ukcrime.health
81   Santry C. NHS trusts criticised over poor complaint
     handling. *Health Service Journal.* 16 February 2009
     11:31.
82   Personal Communication from Tessa Ing, Head of
     'End of Life Care', Department of Health, Room 403
     Wellington House, 133-155 Waterloo Road, London
     SE1 8UG. See also:
     http://www.healthcarecommission.org.uk/
     newsandevents/mediacentre/
     pressreleases.cfm?cit_id=791&FAArea1=customWid
     gets.content_view_1&usecache=false
83   http://www.complaintexpert.co.uk/health-
     complaints.html
84   ibid. http://www.complaintexpert.co.uk/health-
     complaints.html
85   Koenig HG. *Aging and God: spiritual pathways to
     mental health in midlife and later years: using religion to
     cope.* New York.The Haworth Press inc. 1994. p.502.
86   Commission for Healthcare Audit and Inspection.
     *Caring for dignity: a national report on dignity in care
     for older people while in hospital.* 2007.
87   The 'Liverpool Care Pathway' is a continuous

quality improvement framework for care of the dying, irrespective of diagnosis or place of death.

88   Livesley B. The management of the dying patient. In: Pathy MSJ, ed. *Principles and Practice of Geriatric Medicine*. Chichester. J Wiley and Sons Ltd. 1985. pp.1287-1295.

89   This allows events to take a natural course during the appropriate relief and prevention of distressing symptoms. It does *not* invoke inappropriate resuscitation procedures which, without therapeutic benefit, would prolong the individual's suffering and prevent their ability to die naturally. Likewise, it is not to be interpreted as causing the patient's death by the illegal double effect mechanism. For an outline of the philosophical and legal issues see the sections on 'Extraordinary and ordinary means' and 'Intention and motive' in *The New Dictionary of Medical Ethics*. [eds.] Boyd KM, Higgs R, Pinching AJ. BMJ Publishing Group, 1997. pp.93-94, and 137-139, respectively. In this writer's [BL's] opinion the pronouncement by the United States of America's Supreme Court '…that terminal sedation intended for symptomatic relief is not assisted suicide….' is one that clearly distinguishes between conduct to intentionally hasten death and that which is intended to relieve pain or other symptoms. [See: Orentlicher D. [Sounding board] The Supreme Court speaks: not assisted suicide but a constitutional right to palliative care. *The New England Journal of Medicine* 1997; 337(17):1234-1236. Orentlicher points out that '…the principle of double effect justifies only the sedation that is part of terminal sedation. We cannot justify the withdrawal of food and water during terminal sedation, for that step does nothing to relieve that

patient's suffering but only serves to bring about the patient's death. If it is argued that the withdrawal of food and water is a permissible act, then we are back to the previous response that it is permissible only because the patient's inability to eat or drink results from an underlying disease.']

90   Livesley. 1989. op.cit.

91   Henderson R. The decline of the professions and their regulation: Ormrod Lecture given at The Inner Temple on 7 April 2008. *Medicine, Science and the Law* 2008;48(4);277-287.

92   Turner-Warwick M. The patient-doctor relationship over 60 years and the role of the Royal Medical Colleges. *Clinical Medicine* 2008;8(6);573-575.

93   Williamson, J. Doctors and the elderly dying patient. *Geriatric Medicine* 1981;2(8);6-8.

94   'Severn had designed an emblem, a Greek lyre with half its strings broken or untied. … Although Taylor wished only for the words Keats had requested, "Here lies one whose name was writ in water", Brown wanted a preface, "This Grave contains all that was Mortal, of a YOUNG ENGLISH POET Who, on his Death Bed, in the Bitterness of his Heart at the Malicious Power of his Enemies, Desired these Words to be engraven [*sic*] on his Tomb Stone."' The inscription was cut late in the year (1822). See: Scott. op.cit. pp.434-435.

95   http://www.1911encyclopedia.org/Francis_Beaumont_and_John_Fletcher

96   http://www.uq.edu.au/emsah/drama/fletcher/nf/philaster/f2/complete/philaster.htm/_Beaumont F, Fletcher J. [authors] *Philaster: or, Love Lies a Bleeding.* 1679;Act 5;Sc.3; lines 2199-2221.

97   Shakespeare W. *King Henry VIII.* 1611; Act IV: Sc.ii. Griffith's speech.

98 Sanderson (Sir) W. *Art of painting in water colours.* 1658 [cited by Hebb J. Keats's epitaph on himself. Notes and queries. 1898 (September 3) 9th S.II: p.186].

99 Kipling R. *Something of myself for my friends known and unknown.* Macmillan & Co, Limited. London. 1937. pp.208-210. See also: Bromwich D. Kipling's Jest. *Grand Street* 1985; 4(2);150-179.

100 Tompkins JMS. *The art of Rudyard Kipling.* University Paperbacks. 1965. p.94.

101 Kipling R. *Wireless.* First published in *Scribner's Magazine,* August 1902, and collected in *Traffic and discoveries* in 1904 and subsequently in several other editions of the same title. This writer's copy is the 1949 edition published by Macmillan and Co., Ltd. London. In this story Kipling writes of the early days of the wireless telegraph. It concerns a chemist [apothecary], who has tuberculosis and drugged himself and, who although never having read Keats, he is decribed by Kipling as writing several lines of Keats' poem 'The Eve of St. Agnes'. Kipling suggests this ability resulted from his picking up Keats' 'universal spiritual vibrations'.

102 Carrington C. *Rudyard Kipling: his life and work.* London. Macmillan & co Ltd. 1955. p.421.

103 ibid. pp.352-356.

104 Fischer SR. *A history of writing.* Reaktion Books Ltd. 2005. p.295.

105 Personal communication.

106 Keats J. [author] Letter to Fanny Brawne, Tuesday morn, May (?) 1820. Scott. op.cit. pp.442-443.

107 Poel JVD. *The Jameson Raid.* London. Oxford University Press. 1951.

108 Kipling R. 1904. op.cit. p.94.

109 Kipling R. *Rewards and fairies.* Macmillan and Co.,

Ltd. London. 1910. pp.175-176.

[110] 'A Doctor of Medicine' is written around Nicholas Culpeper and an outbreak of plague; and, 'Marklake Witches' is written around Réne Laennec's discovery of the stethoscope. These two stories appear to compare the old and new styles of medical practice. In another of the stories, entitled 'Wrong Thing', a psychological problem, involving recurring thoughts of inferiority and hatred, is resolved and also helps to convey the theme of healing in *Rewards and Fairies*.

[111] Livesley B. New aspects of William Osler? (1849–1919). Lecture to the Medical Society of London. 233rd Session, 2005-2006. Presented at a special joint meeting with the Osler Club of London. 13th February 2006.

[112] ibid.

[113] Osler Sir W. The evolution of internal medicine [in] *A System of Medicine*. [ed.] Osler W, McCrae T. 1907;1:xxxiv. London. Oxford University Press.